Pescatarian Diet Cookbook

Easy, Delicious Pescatarian and Vegetarian Recipes for a Balanced Lifestyle

Jacob Aiello

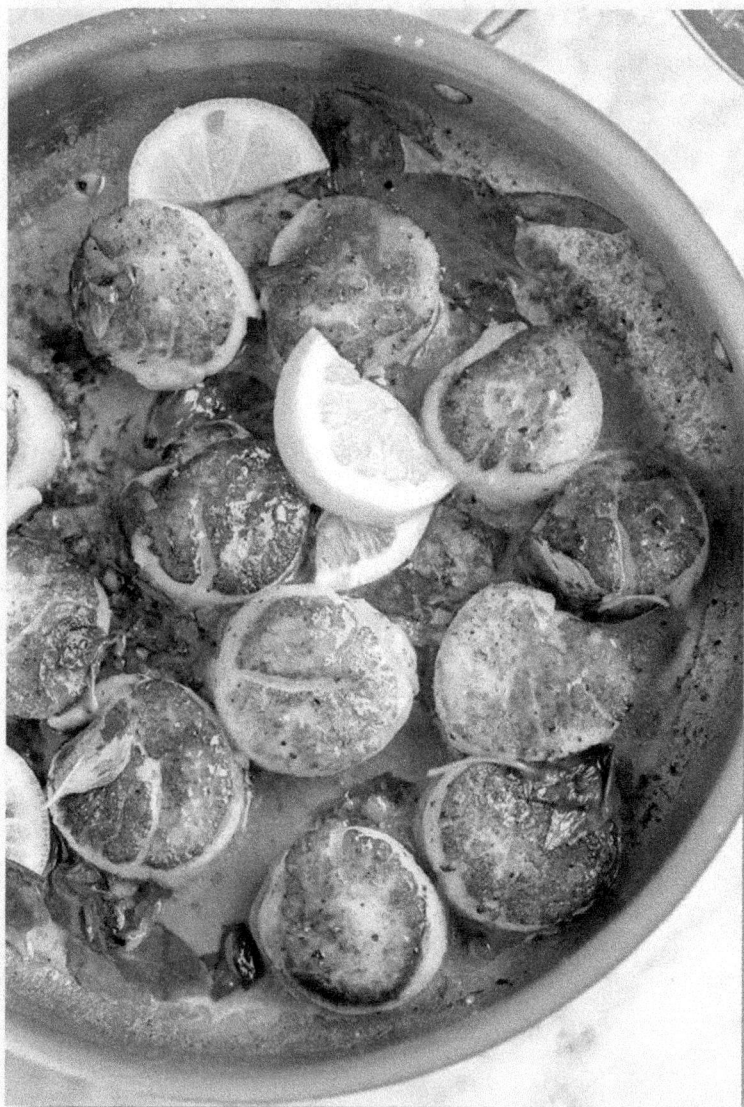

Table of Contents

VEGETARIAN RECIPES

The vegetarian recipes in this cookbook were inspired by the Mediterranean lifestyle, which helps you cook delicious meals with healthy, locally available ingredients that you can buy or even grow in your backyard. Some of the commonly used ingredients in these vegetarian recipes include: extra virgin olive oil, fresh vegetables, protein-rich legumes, nuts, seeds, healthy cheeses, aromatic, super food herbs and spices.

All Mediterranean vegetarian dishes are generally prepared slowly in an all-in-one pot and are very rarely fried. Another benefit of vegetarian meal is that they usually have low WW food point scores, most of the dishes even have zero point score. This helps you achieve your weight loss set target within the possible shortest period of time. Not only that, you will also enjoy delicious meals while still meeting your healthy lifestyle and weight loss target. The meals in this cookbook will keep you free from digestion problems, excess weight gain, diabetes and also keep you free from heart diseases.

You will find in this cookbook, delicious vegetarian soups and salads recipes that can serve as main meal, side dish or even use it to garnish your seafood dishes.

VEGETARIAN SALADS

Zucchini Salad with Greek Yogurt

Servings: 4

Ingredients and Quantity

- 3 medium zucchinis, coarsely chopped
- 1 cup Greek Yogurt
- 1/2 cup walnuts, crushed
- 2 garlic cloves, chopped
- 2 tbsp. extra virgin olive oil
- 1 tsp. paprika
- 1 tbsp. dried mint
- 1/2 cup fresh dill, finely cut
- Salt, to taste

Direction

1. Grate the zucchinis and squeeze them with your hands to drain excessive juice.

2. Heat the olive oil in a pan and gently cook zucchinis, stirring, for 4 to 5 minutes or until tender.

3. Stir in paprika and set aside to cool down.

4. When zucchinis have cooled down, add in garlic, walnuts, dill, mint and salt. Stir to combine well and add in yogurt.

5. Stir again. Best served cold. Enjoy!

Cucumber Salad

Servings: 4

Ingredients and Quantity

- 2 medium cucumbers, peeled and sliced
- A bunch fresh dill
- 2 to 3 cloves garlic, pressed
- 3 tbsp. white wine vinegar
- 3 tbsp. olive oil
- Salt, to taste

Direction

1. Cut the cucumbers in rings and put them in a salad bowl.
2. Add the finely cut dill, the pressed garlic and season with salt, vinegar and oil.
3. Toss to combine. Best served cold. Enjoy!

Carrot Salad with Yogurt

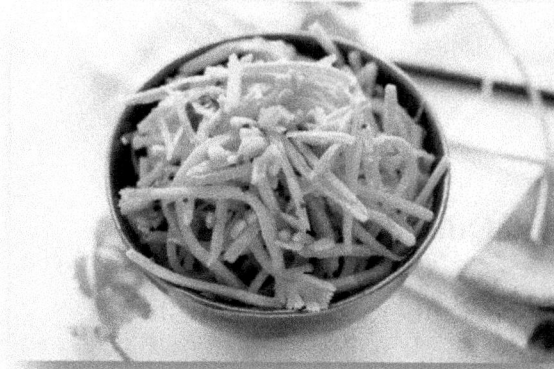

Servings: 4

Ingredients and Quantity

- 4 to 5 carrots, grated
- 3 garlic cloves, pressed
- 1/2 cup Greek yogurt
- 2 tbsp. mayonnaise
- 2 tbsp. olive oil
- 2 tbsp. finely chopped fresh dill
- Salt and pepper, to taste

Direction

1. Heat olive oil in a skillet and gently sauté carrots for 2 to 3 minutes or until wilted.

2. In a bowl, combine carrots, yogurt, mayonnaise, garlic and dill.

3. Add salt and black pepper to your taste.

4. Toss to combine. Serve and enjoy!

Strained Yogurt Salad

Servings: 4

Ingredients and Quantity

- 1 large or 2 small cucumbers, fresh or pickled
- 4 cups yogurt
- 2 to 3 crushed walnuts
- 1/2 bunch dill
- 3 tbsp. sunflower oil
- Salt, to taste

Direction

1. Strain the yogurt in a piece of cheesecloth or a clean white dishtowel.

2. You can suspend it over a bowl or the sink.

3. Peel and dice the cucumbers, place in a large bowl.

4. Add the crushed walnuts and the crushed garlic, the oil and the finely chopped dill.

5. Scoop the drained yogurt into the bowl and stir well.

6. Add salt to the taste, cover with cling film and put in the fridge for at least an hour so that the flavors can mix well. Serve and enjoy!

Turkish Beet Salad with Yogurt

Servings: 4

Ingredients and Quantity

- 3 medium beet roots
- 1 cup strained yogurt
- 1 garlic clove, minced
- 1 tsp. white vinegar or lemon juice
- 1 tbsp. extra virgin olive oil
- 1/4 tsp. dried mint
- 1/2 tsp. salt

Direction

1. Wash the beets well, cut the stems and steam in a pot or pan for 25 to 30 minutes or until properly cooked.

2. When they cool down, pat dry with paper towel.

3. Grate beets and put them in a deep bowl.

4. Add the other ingredients and toss. Best served cold.

   Enjoy!

Spinach Stem Salad

Servings: 2

Ingredients and Quantity

- Few bunches of spinach stems
- Water, for boiling the stems
- 1 garlic clove, minced
- Lemon juice or vinegar, to taste
- Extra virgin olive oil
- Salt, to taste

Direction

1. Trim the stems so that they will remain intact.

2. Wash the stems very well.

3. Steam the stems in a basket over boiling water for 2 to 3 minutes until wilted but not too fluffy.

4. Place them in a plate and sprinkle with minced garlic, olive oil, lemon juice or vinegar and salt. Serve and enjoy!

Roasted Eggplant and Pepper Relish

Servings: 4

Ingredients and Quantity

- 2 medium sized eggplants
- 2 red or green bell peppers
- 2 tomatoes
- 3 garlic cloves, crushed
- Some fresh parsley
- 1 to 2 tbsp. red wine vinegar
- Extra virgin oil, to taste
- Salt and pepper, to taste

Direction

1. Wash and dry the vegetables.
2. Prick the skin of the eggplants.

3. Bake the eggplants, tomatoes and peppers in a pre-heated oven at 400 F for about 40 minutes, until the skins are pretty burnt.

4. Take out of the oven and leave in a covered container for about 10 minutes.

5. Peel the skins off and drain well the extra juices.

6. De-seed the peppers.

7. Cut all the vegetables into small pieces.

8. Add the garlic and mix well with a fork or in a food processor.

9. Add the olive oil, vinegar and salt to taste. Stir again.

10. Serve cold and sprinkle parsley on top. Enjoy!

Kale Salad with Creamy Tahini Dressing

Servings: 4

Ingredients and Quantity

- 1 head kale
- 2 cucumbers, peeled and diced
- 1 avocado, peeled and diced
- 1 red onion, finely chopped
- 1 cup cherry tomatoes, halved

For the Dressing:

- 1/3 cup tahini
- /2 cup water
- garlic cloves, minced
- 3 tbsp. lemon juice
- 4 tbsp. extra virgin olive oil
- Salt and freshly ground black pepper, to taste

Direction

1. Prepare the dressing by whisking all ingredients.

2. Place all salad ingredients in a bowl and toss with the dressing.

3. Season to taste with black pepper and salt. Serve and enjoy!

Brown Lentil Salad

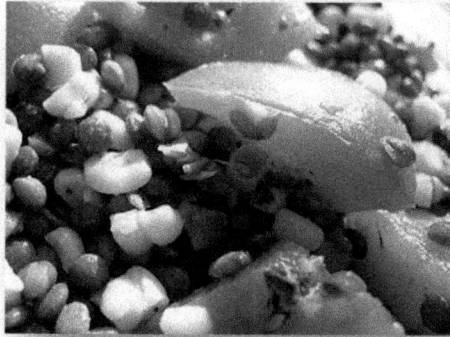

Servings: 4

Ingredients and Quantity

- 1 can lentils, drained and rinsed
- 1 red onion, thinly sliced
- 1 tomato, diced
- 1 red bell pepper, chopped
- 2 garlic cloves, crushed
- 2 tbsp. lemon juice
- 1/3 cup parsley leaves
- Salt and pepper, to taste

Direction

1. Place lentils, red onion, tomatoes, bell pepper and lemon juice in a large bowl.

2. Season with salt and black pepper to taste.

3. Toss to combine and sprinkle with parsley. Serve and enjoy!

Bulgur with Walnuts and Green Lentils

Servings: 4

Ingredients and Quantity

- 1 cup bulgur
- 1 cup hot water
- 1/2 cup cooked green lentils
- 1/2 cup walnuts, crushed
- 1 cup halved cherry tomatoes
- 1 red or green, pepper, cut
- 3 to 4 spring onion, finely cut
- /2 cup parsley, finely cut
- 1 tbsp. dried mint
- 1 tsp. dried basil
- 3 tbsp. extra virgin olive oil
- Salt and pepper, to taste

Direction

1. In a bowl, combine bulgur, hot water and olive oil.

2. Stir, cover and set aside for 15 minutes to steam.

3. Add in lentils, walnuts, onions, pepper, tomatoes and salt to your taste.

4. Also add the parsley, dried basil and mint.

5. Toss to combine. Serve and enjoy!

Slimming Ginger Steamed Fish

Preparation time: 20 Minutes

Ingredients

- 1/2 red pepper julienned
- 1 large clove garlic sliced thinly
- 1 tablespoon soy sauce
- 1/2 tablespoon mirin
- 1 tablespoon sesame oil
- 1/2 tsp. Thai chili deseeded and sliced very thin
- 2 5oz fillets halibut or other white fish
- 1 tsp. Salt
- 3 scallions julienned
- 2 tablespoon ginger julienned

Directions

1. Place one of the fillets in a heatproof bowl that will fit in your steamer, and top with half of the salt, scallions, ginger, red peppers and garlic.

2. Place another fillet on top of the first and repeat the process with the remaining ingredients.

3. Add the chili, soy sauce, and mirin and sesame oil.

4. Put 1 inch of water in the bottom a pot over medium heat and place steamer in the pot.

5. Place the bowl with the fish in the steamer (the water should not be touching the steamer or the bowl) and cover the pot.

6. Steam the fish for 15-20 minutes depending on the thickness of your fillets.

7. Serve with brown rice and half a lemon.

One Pan Baked Teriyaki Salmon

Preparation time: 30 Minutes

Ingredients

- 1/2 lb. salmon fillet
- 2 zucchini cut into small cubes
- 2 carrots cut into 2 small cubes
- 1 tablespoon salt course
- 1 1/2 tablespoon sesame oil
- 2 tablespoon scallions chopped (green parts only)
- 1 tablespoon sesame seeds
- 1 tablespoon ginger peeled and cut into matchsticks
- 2 cloves garlic
- 1/2 tablespoon corn starch
- 2/3 cup pineapple cubed
- 1/2 orange sliced into 6 slices
- 1/2 cup soy sauce
- 1/4 cup mirin

- 2 tablespoon maple syrup

- 1/2 orange juiced

Directions

1. Pre-heat oven to 400°F.

2. In a pot over medium heat, combine the soy sauce, mirin, orange juice and bring to a boil. Reduce heat and add the pineapple and stir until thick.

3. Lay the salmon fillet skin side down on a baking sheet covered in parchment paper and slide the orange under the fillet halfway. Surround the outside of the fillet with the zucchini and carrot.

4. Season with salt and the sesame oil and pour the marinade on top of the salmon fillet saving a little to dress the dish at the end.

5. Bake for 15 minutes then broil for 5 minutes or until the top is caramelized, then garnish with more sauce, scallions and sesame seeds. Serve and enjoy!

Blackened Fish Tacos with Cabbage Mango Slaw

Preparation time: 45 Minutes

Ingredients

For Tacos:

- 1 lb. skinless cod or halibut filet
- 1/2 lime, juiced
- Cooking spray
- 8 corn tortillas
- Lime wedges for serving
- 1/2 lime, cut into wedges
- 1/4 tsp. (1/2 tsp. for spicier) ground cayenne pepper
- 1/4 tsp. ground cumin
- 1/4 tsp. ground oregano
- 1/8 tsp. black pepper
- 1 tsp. smoked paprika
- 1 tsp. kosher salt
- ½ tsp. dry mustard

For Cabbage Slaw:

- 3 1/2 cups (1/2 small) red cabbage, shredded fine
- 1 mango, julienned
- 2 tsp. olive oil
- 1/4 cup cilantro
- 1/2 tsp. kosher salt
- 1 lime, juiced

Directions

1. Combine all the slaw ingredients and refrigerate.

2. In a small bowl, mix the dried spices and seasoning together, squeeze the lime on the fish then rub the seasoning onto fish.

3. On grill or stove on high heat, heat a cast iron skillet till really hot. Spray with nonstick oil spray.

4. Cook fish for about 5mins on each side until opaque in the center and well browned on the outside. Heat the corn tortillas on the grill for about 1 to 2 minutes or until they slightly char.

5. Cut the fish into 8 pieces (or you can flake it if it's easier).

6. Divide the fish equally between 8 tortillas and top each with 1/2 cup slaw. Serve with lime wedges.

Garlic Lemon Scallops

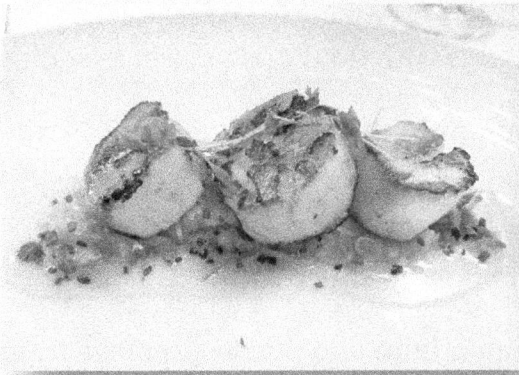

Preparation time: 30 Minutes

Ingredients

- 1 pinch ground sage
- 1 lemon, juiced
- 2 tbsp. parsley, chopped
- 1 lb. scallops
- 2 tbsps. All-purpose flour
- 1 tbsp. olive oil
- 4 garlic cloves, minced
- 1 scallion, finely chopped

Directions

1. Heat the oil in a large non- stick skillet.

2. Toss scallops with flour and salt, in a medium bowl

3. Place scallops in the skillet; add garlic, scallions, and sage.

4. Sauté for about 3-4hrs or until scallops are just opaque

5. Stir in lemon juice and parsley; remove from heat and serve immediately.

Shrimp & Broccoli in Chili Sauce

Preparation: 95 Minutes

Ingredients

- 2 teaspoon corn starch
- 2 teaspoon sugar
- 1⁄2 teaspoon salt
- 1 tablespoon oil
- 3 cup broccoli, cut into florets
- 4 cup cooked soba noodles,
- 8 oz. uncooked buckwheat noodles, or vermicelli
- 2 tablespoons dry sherry
- 1 1/2 teaspoons paprika
- 1/2 teaspoon ground red pepper
- 4 garlic cloves, crushed
- 1/3 cup water
- 1/4 cup chili sauce (like Heinz)
- 2 lb. medium shrimp, peeled and deveined
- 2 tablespoons minced seeded jalapeño pepper (about 2 peppers)

Directions

1. In a medium bowl, combine shrimp, jalapeno pepper, sherry, paprika, red pepper and garlic cloves and chill for 1 hour

2. Combine water, chili sauce, corn starch, sugar, salt and oil in another bowl and set aside.

3. Heat oil in a stir fry pan. Add Broccoli and stir fry for 2mins.

4. Add shrimp mixture, stir fry 5 minutes or until shrimp are done, then add cornstarch mixture and bring to a boil. Cook for 1 minute or until sauce thickens.

5. Serve over soba noodles.

Prawn Pitta Scoops

Preparation time: 10 Minutes

Ingredients

- Juice of ½ lemon
- 2 tablespoon fresh coriander leaves
- 160 g (5½ oz.) cooked, peeled prawns
- ½ tsp. paprika
- Salt and freshly ground black pepper to season
- 125g (4¼ oz.) avocado, peeled, stoned and finely chopped
- 200g (7 oz.) tomatoes, quartered, deseeded and finely chopped
- ½ small red onion, finely chopped
- 4 pitta breads

Directions

1. Preheat the grill to high.

2. Meanwhile, open out the Pitta Breads and slice each half in 2 to make 16 pitta scoops.

3. Place on a grill pan, and grill for 4-5 minutes or until golden and toasted.

4. Combine the chopped avocado, tomatoes, onion, lemon juice and coriander and season.

5. Divide the avocado mix between the pitta scoops. Top with the prawns and a pinch of paprika.

6. Serve!

Shrimp with Cilantro and Lime

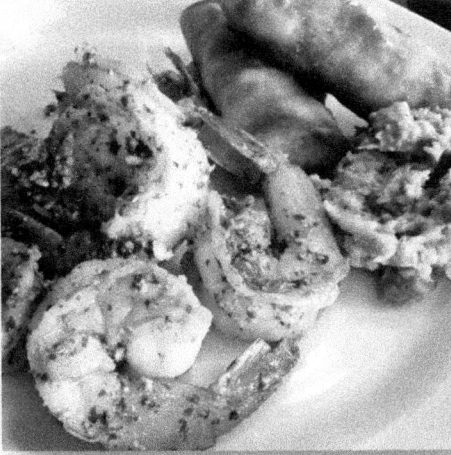

Preparation time: 40 Minutes

Ingredients

- 1 1/2 pounds peeled and deveined jumbo shrimp
- 2 tablespoons lime juice (from 1 medium lime)
- 2 garlic cloves, crushed
- 3 to 4 tablespoons chopped fresh cilantro
- 1 tablespoon olive oil
- 1 teaspoon lime, zest
- Salt and pepper, to taste

Directions

1. In a large bowl, combine shrimp, lime juice, cumin, ginger, and garlic. Toss well.

3. Heat oil in a large nonstick skillet over medium-high heat.

4. Add shrimp mixture and sauté until shrimp is done, about 4mins

5. Remove from heat and stir in cilantro, lime zest, salt, and pepper.

6. Serve!

Maple Mustard Salmon

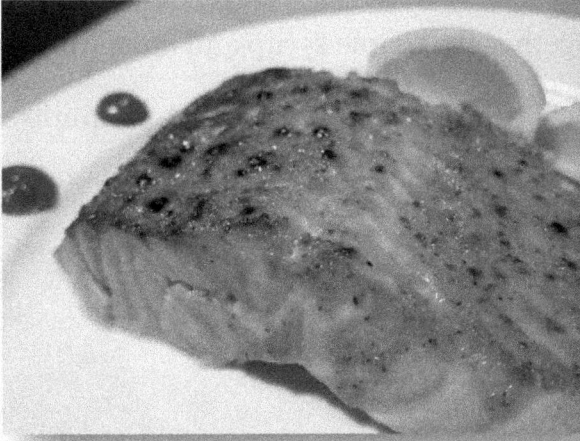

Servings: 4

Ingredients

- 2 tbsp. maple syrup (pure)
- Salt and pepper
- 1.33 lb. raw wild salmon
- 3 tbsp. whole grain mustard

Directions

1. Preheat the oven to 350 degrees F.

2. Mix together the maple syrup and mustard.

3. Brush over the salmon. Bake for 10-12 minutes until cooked to your liking.

Grilled Shrimp Marinade with Shrimp Sauce

Servings: 5

Ingredients

- ½ teaspoon salt
- ½ teaspoon pepper
- Pinch of red pepper flakes

For Sauce:

- 1 tablespoon prepared horseradish sauce
- 2 tablespoons ketchup
- 1 tablespoon non-fat plain Greek yogurt
- 24 medium Shrimp cleaned and deveined
- 2 teaspoons balsamic vinegar
- 1 teaspoon olive oil
- Juice of 1 lemon
- 1 clove garlic minced

Directions

1. In a medium bowl, mix together vinegar, oil, lemon juice, garlic, salt, pepper, and pepper flakes in a medium bowl.

2. Pour over shrimp then covers and refrigerate for a minimum of half an hour.

3. Slide shrimp onto skewers.

4. Grill for 2-3 minutes on each side. Shrimp cooks fast, so watch for it to curl and turn pink.

For Sauce:

1. In a small bowl, mix together all ingredients.

2. Add more or less horseradish sauce to taste

Mexi' Shrimp Salad Wrap

Servings: 4

Ingredients

- 1/2 cup finely chopped romaine lettuce
- 3 tbsp. fresh salsa or pico de gallo
- 2 tbsp. canned black beans, drained and rinsed
- 2 tbsp. frozen corn kernels, thawed
- 2 tbsp. chopped fresh cilantro
- 1 medium-large high-fiber flour tortilla with 110 calories or less
- 2 tbsp. fat-free sour cream
- 1/2 tbsp. fresh lime juice
- 1/8 tsp. ground cumin
- 2 dashes chili powder, or more to taste
- 3 oz. cooked and chopped shrimp

Directions

1. Mix sour cream, lime juice, cumin, chili powder and, if you like, a dash of salt in a large bowl. Stir in all remaining ingredients except tortilla.

2. Spoon mixture across the center of the tortilla.

3. Wrap tortilla up by first folding one side in (to keep filling from escaping), and then tightly rolling it up from the bottom. Enjoy!

Fish and Shrimp Stew

Servings: 4

Ingredients

- 8 oz. clam juice
- 14 oz. fish stock
- 2 tbsp. almond butter (or ghee for Whole 30)
- 1/2 tsp. oregano
- 1/2 tsp. Basil
- Salt and pepper
- 1 tbsp. olive oil
- 1 onion, diced
- 2 garlic cloves, minced
- 1/4 tsp. red pepper flakes (optional, I used double, that's for a spicier soup)
- 2/3 cup parsley
- 3 tbsp. tomato paste
- 28 oz. canned San Marzano tomatoes

Directions

1. Heat the olive oil over medium heat. Add the onion and cook for 5-7 minutes until beginning to become translucent.

2. Add the garlic and red pepper flakes. Cook for 1-2 minutes, stirring often. Add the parsley and cook for 1-2 minutes. Stir in the tomato paste and cook for 1 minute.

3. Add the tomatoes, clam juice, and fish stock. Bring to a simmer and add the butter, oregano, and basil. Simmer for 10-15 minutes. At this point, you want to taste the broth and adjust the seasoning as needed.

4. Add salt and pepper. If needed, add extra tomato paste for more tomato flavor. You can add red pepper flakes for more heat or some extra tomatoes if it is too spicy.

5. Make sure the broth is simmering and add the cod. Cook for 5 minutes. Then add the shrimp and cook for 4-5 minutes until opaque and cooked through.

Skinny Southern BBQ Shrimp

Servings: 4

Ingredients

- 1/4 teaspoon cayenne
- 2 tablespoons Worcestershire sauce
- 1 teaspoon paprika
- 2 teaspoons dried oregano
- 2 teaspoons dried thyme leaves
- Salt and pepper to taste
- 1 pound medium to large peeled shrimp
- 1/3 cup white wine or cooking wine
- 2 tablespoons olive oil
- 2 tablespoons fat-free Caesar or Creamy Italian dressing
- 1 tablespoon minced garlic

Directions

1. Combine oil, Italian dressing, garlic, cayenne,
   Worcestershire sauce, paprika, oregano, thyme, salt and

pepper in large nonstick skillet over medium heat until sauce begins to boil.

2. Add shrimp and cook for 3 to 4 minutes, stirring continuously. Add wine and cook until the shrimp are done, 3 to 5 additional minutes. Serve hot.

Shrimp 'n Slaw Marinara

Servings: 1

Ingredients

- 1/2 cup low-fat marinara sauce
- 4 oz. ready-to-eat shrimp
- One 12-oz. bag (4 cups) broccoli cole slaw
- *For Seasoning:* garlic powder, onion powder, red pepper flakes

Directions

1. Spray a large skillet with nonstick spray to medium-high heat.

2. Add broccoli slaw and 1/2 cup water.

3. Cover and cook until fully softened, about 10 minutes. Uncover and, if needed, cook and stir until water has evaporated, 2 - 3 minutes.

4. Add marinara sauce and shrimp.

5. Cook and stir until hot and well mixed, about 2 minutes. Season to taste!

Cranberry Tuna Salad

Servings: 5

Ingredients

- 1/4 cup red onion, minced
- 1 tbsp. lemon juice
- 1/4 cup dried cranberries
- 1 apple, diced
- Salt and pepper
- 16 oz. can white tuna, packed in water, drained
- 3 tbsp. low fat mayonnaise
- 3 tbsp. light sour cream
- 1/2 cup celery, chopped

Directions

1. Combine all the ingredients. Season with salt and pepper
2. Serve right away!
3. Refrigerate if not eating right away.

England Fish Chowder Recipe

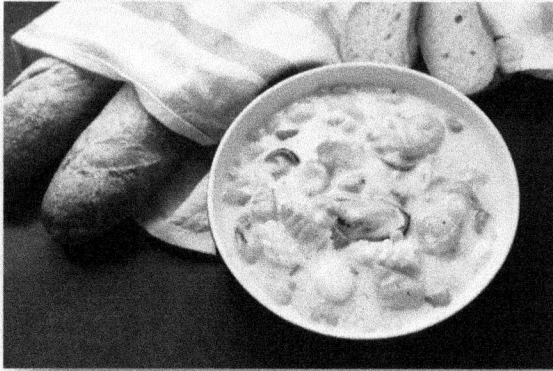

Servings: 3

Ingredients

- 1 teaspoon paprika
- 2 teaspoons dried oregano
- 2 teaspoons dried thyme leaves
- Salt and pepper to taste
- 1 pound medium to large peeled shrimp
- 1/3 cup white wine or cooking wine
- 2 tablespoons olive oil
- 2 tablespoons fat-free Caesar or Creamy Italian dressing
- 1 tablespoon minced garlic

- 1/4 teaspoon cayenne
- 2 tablespoons Worcestershire sauce

Directions

1. Combine oil, Italian dressing, garlic, cayenne, Worcestershire sauce, paprika, oregano, thyme, salt and pepper in large nonstick skillet over medium heat until sauce begins to boil.

2. Add shrimp and cook for 3 to 4 minutes, stirring continuously.

3. Add wine and cook until the shrimp are done, 3 to 5 additional minutes. Serve hot.

Spicy Baked Shrimp

Ingredients

- 2 tsp. low-sodium soy sauce
- Pinch of cayenne pepper
- 1 lb. large shrimp, peeled and deveined
- Lemon wedges
- 1/2 cup olive oil
- 2 tablespoons Cajun seasoning
- 2 tablespoons fresh lemon juice
- 2 tablespoons chopped fresh parsley
- 1 tablespoon maple syrup

Directions

1. Preheat oven to 450 degrees F (230 degrees C).

2. Coat an 11 x 7-inch baking dish with cooking spray.

3. Mix maple syrup, olive oil, dried parsley, cayenne pepper, Cajun seasoning, lemon juice, and soy sauce in dish

4. Add shrimp and toss to coat.

5. Bake for 8 minutes or until shrimp turn pink, stirring occasionally. Garnish with lemon wedges

6. Serve!

Maple Glazed Salmon with Wasabi

Preparation time: 40 Minutes

Ingredients

- 1 lb. salmon fillet, cut into 4 equal pieces
- 1/2 cup Mirin (Japanese sweet rice wine)
- 1 tsp. fresh ginger, peeled and minced
- 2 tablespoons soy sauce
- 1 tbsp. honey
- 2 tsp. wasabi, paste
- 1 tbsp. seasoned rice vinegar
- Salt to taste
- 2 tsp. wasabi, paste
- 1 tablespoon finely grated peeled fresh ginger
- ¼ cup scallion, thinly sliced
- ½ tsp. pepper

Directions

1. Bring vinegar, maple syrup, ginger, mirin, soy sauce, and wasabi to boil in a small saucepan, to make sauce

2. Cook, stirring occasionally, over medium-high heat until the flavors are blended and the sauce is thickened, about 5 minutes.

3. Remove from the heat and cover. Ensure it is kept warm

4. Sprinkle salmon with salt and pepper.

5. Spray a large nonstick skillet with nonstick spray and set over high heat.

6. Add salmon and cook for about 4 minutes on each side, turning once, or until the fish is browned on the outside and opaque in the center.

7. Spoon sauce over the salmon. Sprinkle with scallions and serve.

Walleye Vegetarian Delight

Servings: 4

Calories: 600

Fat: 33.4 g

Protein: 32.8 g

Carbs: 43.8 g

Ingredients and Quantity

- 4 walleye fillets
- 1/2 tbsp. lemon juice
- 1/2 cup white wine
- 1/2 tbsp. orange juice
- 1/8 cup almond butter

For the Vegetable Stuffing:

- 1/2 cup onion, chopped
- 1/4 carrots, thinly sliced
- 1/2 celery, chopped
- 1/2 green pepper, chopped

- 1/4 cup almond butter
- 1 cup seasoned bread crumbs
- 1 cup diced tomato
- 1/8 tsp. salt
- 1/8 tsp. pepper

Direction

1. Place the fillets on a well-greased shallow baking pan.

2. Drizzle with lemon and orange juice.

3. Cover with vegetable stuffing, wine and several slices of butter.

4. Cover with foil and bake at 350 degrees F for 20 minutes.

5. Uncover and continue to bake for 10 to 15 minutes or until fish flakes apart easily with a fork.

6. For the vegetable stuffing; sauté onion, carrots, celery and green pepper in butter until tender, about 10 minutes.

7. Add the remaining ingredients and mix well. Serve and enjoy!

Fish Stuffed Green Pepper

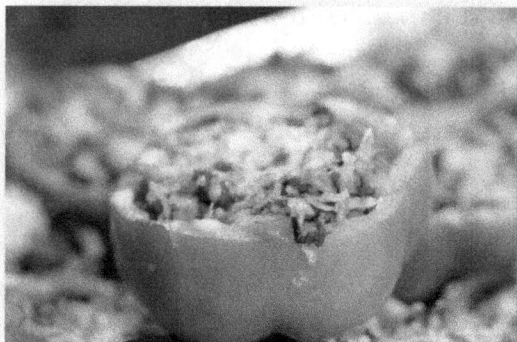

Servings: 4

Calories: 272

Fat: 14.5 g

Protein: 12.5 g

Carbs: 24.4 g

Ingredients and Quantity

- 2 large green peppers
- 2 tbsp. almond butter
- 2 tbsp. flour
- 1/4 tbsp. salt

- Dash pepper
- 1 cup coconut milk
- 1 cup cooked, flaked walleye, yellow perch or other fish
- 1/3 cup celery, chopped
- 1/4 cup bread crumbs

Direction

1. Cut green peppers in half, remove seeds and set aside.
2. Melt butter in a saucepan over low heat.
3. Mix in flour, salt and a dash of pepper. Add milk.
4. Cook over moderate heat, stirring constantly, until mixture thickens.
5. Remove from heat and add fish and celery.
6. Pour mixture into halved green peppers.
7. Top with bread crumbs.
8. Bake at 400 degrees F for 15 minutes. Serve and enjoy!

Oriental Fish with Sweet and Sour Vegetable

Servings: 4

Calories: 748

Fat: 31.8 g

Protein: 36 g

Carbs: 82 g

Ingredients and Quantity

- 2 lb. fish fillets, any firm fleshed fish
- 1 tbsp. lemon juice
- 1 tbsp. vegetable oil
- 2 cups julienne cut carrots
- 1/2 cup onion, thinly sliced
- 2 tbsp. water
- 2 cups sliced celery
- 1/2 cup sliced water chestnuts
- 1 can (8 1/4 oz.) pineapple chunks
- 1 1/2 tbsp. brown sugar

- 3 tbsp. cider vinegar
- 1 1/2 tbsp. soy sauce
- 1 1/2 tbsp. cornstarch

Direction

1. Place fish fillets in a skillet with enough boiling water to barely cover them. Then add lemon juice.
2. Cover and simmer for 8 to 10 minutes until fish flakes apart easily with a fork.
3. Meanwhile, heat vegetable oil in another skillet.
4. Add carrots and onions, stir fry for 5 minutes over moderately high heat.
5. Reduce to moderate heat, add water, cover and steam for 4 minutes.
6. Uncover, add celery and water chestnuts, stir fry for two minutes.
7. Add undrained pineapple.

8. Stir sugar, vinegar, soy sauce and cornstarch slowly into skillet while cooking.

9. Stir until sauce coats vegetables and pineapple.

10. Remove fish from liquid, drain well.

11. Serve topped with sweet-sour vegetable mixture. Enjoy!

Lake Erie Grill-Out

Servings: 6

Calories: 459

Fat: 27.8 g

Protein: 22.6 g

Carbs: 32.1 g

Ingredients and Quantity

- 2 lb. fish fillets (walleye, smallmouth bass or freshwater drum) 1/2 cup
- 3 tbsp. lemon juice
- 3 tbsp. liquid smoke
- 2 tbsp. Vinegar
- 1 tbsp. Salt
- 2 tbsp. Worcestershire sauce
- 1/2 tbsp. grated onion
- 1 clove garlic, finely chopped or 1 tablespoon garlic powder
- 3 drops hot pepper or Tabasco sauce (optional)

Direction

1. Cut fillets into serving size pieces.

2. Place in single layer in shallow baking dish.

3. In a separate bowl, combine remaining ingredients.

4. Pour half the mixture over fillets and marinade for 45 minutes in refrigerator, turn once.

5. Remove fish and place in a hinged wire grill.

6. Use the other half of marinade for basting.

7. Cook 4 inches from medium hot coals for 8, basting frequently.

8. Turn, baste again and cook 7 to10 minutes longer or until fish flakes apart easily with a fork

Fish Hash

Servings: 2

Calories: 529

Fat: 33.6 g

Protein: 21.7 g

Carbs: 38.3 g

Ingredients and Quantity

- 1 cup cold cooked fish fillets
- 1 cup cold boiled potatoes
- 1 large onion, grated
- 1/4 tsp. sage
- 1 egg, beaten
- 3 tbsp. almond butter
- Minced parsley, green onions or ketchup, for serving

Direction

1. Cut the sweet potatoes into small pieces and flake the fish.

2. Add onion, sage and beaten egg.

3. Melt butter in a large frying pan.

4. When hot, press the hash in and cook over medium heat until crusty brown underneath.

5. Invert on to a hot platter and sprinkle to taste with minced parsley, green onions or ketchup. Serve and enjoy!

Fish Burgers

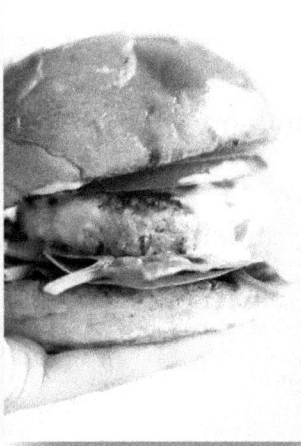

Servings: 2

Calories: 375

Fat: 22.1 g

Protein: 17.8 g

Carbs: 26 g

Ingredients and Quantity

- 1 lb. ground fish
- 1 tbsp. lemon juice

- 1/4 cup flour
- 1/2 tsp. Salt
- 1/8 tsp. pepper
- 1/2 vegetable oil
- 6 split, heated hamburger buns
- 6 lettuce leaves
- 2 tbsp. vegan mayonnaise
- 6 tomato slices

Direction

1. Sprinkle ground fish with lemon juice.

2. Mix flour, salt and pepper.

3. Cover the fish with the flour mixture.

4. Panfry in 1/4 inch hot oil until burgers are lightly browned.

5. In each bun arrange crisp lettuce, fish patty, mayonnaise and a slice of tomato. Serve and enjoy!

Baked Whole Fish with Mushrooms

Servings: 6

Calories: 686

Fat: 34 g

Protein: 73.4 g

Carbs: 17.8 g

Ingredients and Quantity

- 3 1/2 lb. whole striped bass or rainbow tout
- 1/2 cup flour
- 1/8 tsp. salt
- 1/8 tsp. pepper
- 3 tbsp. extra virgin olive oil
- 2 tbsp. almond butter
- 1 rib celery, thinly sliced
- 1 medium carrot, thinly sliced
- 1 can (8 oz.) mushrooms, thinly sliced
- 1/4 cup parsley, minced

- 2 tbsp. dry white wine
- 1/4 tsp. salt and pepper
- 1 1/3 cups spaghetti sauce with mushrooms
- ¼ cup green onions, sliced Lemon wedges, for garnishing

Direction

1. Coat fish with flour and then sprinkle with 1/8 tsp. salt and pepper.

2. Sauté in oil and butter in large skillet until brown, and then remove it.

3. Sauté celery, carrots, mushrooms, parsley, wine, 1/4 tsp. salt and pepper for 5 minutes.

4. Spread 2/3 of the celery mixture on oven-proof platter and then spoon 2/3 cup sauce over it.

5. Stuff fish with remaining celery mixture and then arrange on platter.

6. Spoon remaining sauce on fish.

7. Bake at 425 degrees F until fish is tender, about 20 minutes.

8. Sprinkle with green onions and then garnish with lemon. Serve and enjoy

Citrus Marinated Fish Fillets

Servings: 2

Calories: 371

Fat: 15.7 g

Protein: 42.7 g

Carbs: 18.7 g

Ingredients and Quantity

- 1 pound fresh or frozen fish fillets
- 2/3 cup lime juice
- 2 tbsp. vegetable oil
- 4 tsp. maple syrup
- 2/3 cup water
- 1 tsp. dried dill weed
- 1/2 tsp. salt

Direction

1. Thaw fish, if frozen.

2. Separate fillets or cut into 4 serving-sized portions.

3. Put fish in a shallow pan.

4. For marinade, mix lime juice, vegetable oil, maple syrup, water, dill weed and salt.

5. Divide marinade into 2 equal portions, reserve and store one portion in refrigerator.

6. Pour the other portion of marinade over the fish.

7. Cover and refrigerate for 3 hours or overnight, turning fish occasionally.

8. Remove fish from the pan, disposing of used marinade.

9. Place fish on slightly greased rack of a broiler pan.

10. Broil fish 4 inches from heat until fish flakes easily when tested with fork, allow 5 minutes for each 1/2-inch thickness.

11. Baste fish often with reserved portion of marinade during broiling. Serve and enjoy!

Southern Bass Chowder

Servings: 4

Calories: 427

Fat: 18.5 g

Protein: 53.6 g

Carbs: 10 g

Ingredients and Quantity

- 1/4 cup almond butter
- 1 tbsp. flour
- 1/2 cup scallions, chopped
- 1 garlic clove, minced
- 1/4 cup green pepper, chopped
- 1/2 cup celery, chopped
- 1/2 cup zucchini, chopped
- 1 can (16 oz.) tomatoes
- 1/2 cup dry sherry
- 1 tbsp. lemon juice
- 3 tbsp. tabasco sauce

- 1/8 tsp. salt and pepper
- 1/2 tbsp. thyme
- 2 lb. bass fillets

Direction

1. Melt the butter in skillet.

2. Blend in flour and stir over heat for 2 minutes.

3. Add scallions, garlic, green pepper, celery and zucchini, and then cook until vegetables are soft.

4. Chop tomatoes into small pieces and add to skillet.

5. Combine all other ingredients except fish, and mix well.

6. Simmer uncovered for 1 1/2 hours, adding a little water if necessary, stirring occasionally.

7. Place fish fillets on top of sauce.

8. Cover and increase heat.

9. Cook for 10 minutes or until fish flakes apart easily with a fork.

10. 10.Serve over rice or grits. Enjoy!

Seasoned Fish

Servings: 9

Calories: 366

Fat: 24.2 g

Protein: 14 g

Carbs: 24.4 g

- **Ingredients and Quantity**
- 1/2 package (6 oz. package) oyster crackers, crushed
- 1/2 tsp. lemon pepper
- 1/2 tsp. seasoned salt
- 1/2 cup vegetable oil
- 1 tsp. dill weed
- envelope (1 oz.) Hidden Valley salad dressing
- 9 fish fillets

Direction

1. Mix together crackers, lemon pepper, salt, oil, dill weed and salad dressing.

2. Preheat oven to 375 degrees F.

3. Pour 1/2 cup oil onto a cookie sheet with sides, until bottom is covered.

4. Put cookie sheet in oven while coating fish.

5. Coat fish fillets with cracker mixture.

6. Put fillets on cookie sheet when oil is hot and return to oven.

7. Turn fillets several times until golden brown, or fry 6 1/2 minutes on each side. Serve and enjoy!

Lemon Fish Roll Ups

Servings: 8

Calories: 377

Fat: 23.7 g

Protein: 18.7 g

Carbs: 23.9 g

Ingredients and Quantity

- 1/3 cup almond butter
- 2 tsp. salt
- 1/3 cup lemon juice
- 1 1/3 cups cooked white rice
- 1 cup sharp cheddar cheese, shredded
- package (10 oz.) frozen broccoli, thawed, chopped
- 8 fish fillets
- Paprika, for topping

Direction

1. In small saucepan, melt butter.

2. Add salt, pepper and lemon juice. Set aside.

3. In medium bowl, combine rice, cheese, broccoli and 1/4 cup of the lemon mixture.

4. Place 1/8th of the rice mixture on top of each of the 8 fish fillets and roll the fillets up.

5. Place seam-side down in 11x7-inch baking dish.

6. Top with remaining sauce, then sprinkle with paprika.

7. Bake at 375 degrees F for 25 minutes or until fish flakes with fork. Serve and enjoy!

Fish in Creole Sauce

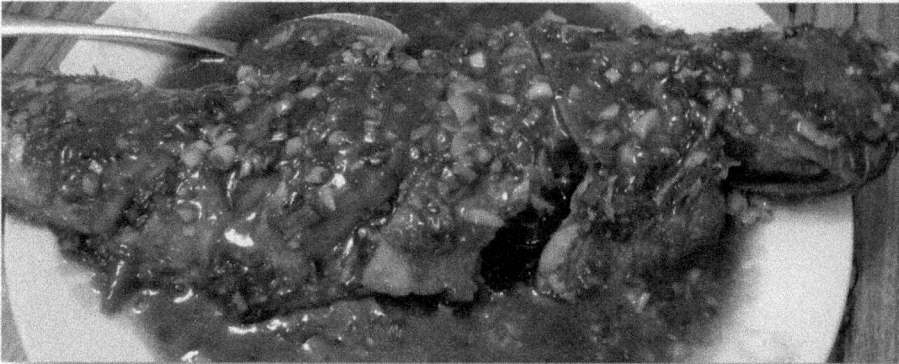

Servings: 6

Calories: 981

Fat: 25.2 g

Protein: 113.8 g

Carbs: 67.1 g

Ingredients and Quantity

- 2 tbsp. almond butter
- 1/4 cup onion, chopped
- 1 garlic clove, minced
- 6 green olives, minced

- 2 cups stewed tomatoes
- 1/2 green pepper, chopped
- 1/2 bay leaf
- 3 beef bouillon cubes
- 1/8 tsp. Thyme
- 2 tsp. parsley, chopped
- 1 tsp. Sugar
- 1/3 tsp. Salt
- Cayenne pepper to taste
- 1/4 cup white wine
- 1/4 cup mushrooms, sliced
- 5 Northern pike fillets, boned and cut in 2 inches chunks
- 25 frozen medium shrimp
- 6 cups cooked rice

Direction

1. Melt the butter and sauté onion, garlic and olives about 2 minutes.

2. Add and cook the rest of the ingredients, except the fillets and shrimp, until sauce is thickened, about 50 minutes.

3. Add fillet chunks and 20 to 25 frozen shrimp to the sauce and cook for 15 minutes or until fish is well cooked.

4. Serve over hot rice. Enjoy!

Easy Fish 'N' Chips

Servings: 4

Calories: 598

Fat: 36.7 g

Protein: 18.9 g

Carbs: 45.3 g

Ingredients and Quantity

- 1/2 cup almond butter
- 2 potatoes, peeled and cut in 1/4 inch slices
- 3/4 cup Ritz crackers, crushed
- 2 tbsp. parsley
- 1 tsp. paprika
- 3/4 tsp. salt
- 1/2 tsp. garlic powder
- 1 lb. frozen fish fillets, thawed

Direction

1. Melt butter 9 by 13 inch pan.

2. Add potato slices and stir to blend.

3. Cover with foil and bake at 350 degrees F for 20 to 25 minutes.

4. Combine crackers, parsley, paprika, salt and garlic powder.

5. Spoon potatoes to one side of baking dish.

6. Dip fillets into melted butter that potatoes were in; then roll in crumb mixture.

7. Place fillets in same baking dish with potatoes.

8. Sprinkle with remaining crumb mixture.

9. Return to oven and continue baking, uncovered for 20 to 30 minutes. Serve and enjoy!

Easy Baked Fillets

Servings: 4

Calories: 277

Fat: 16.2 g

Protein: 14.8 g

Carbs: 19.7 g

Ingredients and Quantity

- 4 fish fillets
- 1 cup shrimp, cooked and deveined
- 4 tbsp. mayonnaise
- 4 slices lemon
- Aluminum foil

Direction

1. Cut 4 large rectangles of aluminum foil.

2. Put one fillet on each rectangle.

3. Add 1/4 cup shrimp on top of each fillet and 1 tbsp. mayonnaise on top of that.

4. Wrap foil around fish tightly and bake at 375 degrees F for 10

5. minutes or until fish flakes easily with fork.

6. Serve with a slice of lemon. Enjoy!

Broiled Fish with Dijon Sauce

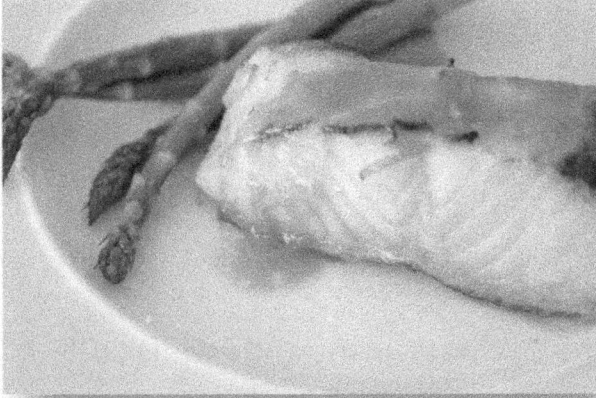

Servings: 3

Calories: 532

Fat: 33.5 g

Protein: 24.9 g

Carbs: 35.8 g

Ingredients and Quantity

- 3 tbsp. vegan cheese, freshly grated
- 2 tbsp. Dijon mustard
- 1/2 cup mayonnaise

- 1/8 tsp. black pepper
- 1 lb. firm fish fillets

Direction

1. In a bowl, mix the cheese, mustard, mayonnaise and pepper.

2. Spread cheese mixture on the fillets.

3. Broil the fillets for 4 to 7 minutes, depending on the size and thickness of the fish, or just until the fish flakes with a fork. Serve and enjoy!

Baked Fish Fillets

Servings: 4

Calories: 383

Fat: 20.1 g

Protein: 18.1 g

Carbs: 34.2 g

Ingredients and Quantity

- 1 lb. fish fillets
- 2 tbsp. lemon juice
- 2 tbsp. almond butter, melted
- 1/4 tsp. dill weed
- 1/2 tsp. Salt
- 1/4 tsp. Pepper
- 2 cups Total cereal, crushed

Direction

1. Grease baking pan.

2. If the fillets are large, cut into serving sizes.

3. Mix lemon juice and butter; reserve.

4. Mix dill weed, salt and pepper.

5. Dip each fillet in butter mixture; sprinkle with salt mixture and coat with cereal.

6. Bake, uncovered, at 350 degrees F for 20 to 30 minutes or until fish flakes easily. Serve and enjoy!

Fillet Almondine

Servings: 4

Calories: 453

Fat: 29.9 g

Protein: 18.5 g

Carbs: 28 g

Ingredients and Quantity

- 1/3 cup almonds, sliced or silvered
- 1/4 cup almond butter
- 1 pound lean fish fillets
- 1/2 tbsp. salt
- 1 tbsp. dry white wine or lemon juice

Direction

1. Place almonds and the butter in a 9-inch pie plate.

2. Microwave on high for 3 to 5 minutes until almonds are golden, stirring twice.

3. Remove almonds with a slotted spoon and set aside.

4. Add fillets to butter, turning to coat.

5. Arrange fillets in dish with thicker portions towards the outside of dish.

6. Cover with wax paper.

7. Microwave on high 4 to 6 minutes, until fish begins to flake when fork is inserted in thickest part.

8. Sprinkle with salt, wine or lemon juice and reserved almonds. Serve and enjoy!

Fish Fillets in Foil

Servings: 4

Calories: 477

Fat: 14.5 g

Protein: 20.3 g

Carbs: 66 g

Ingredients and Quantity

- 4 fillets of fish
- 4 pieces aluminum foil
- 1 cup salsa
- 4 cups hot cooked white rice
- Lime wedges, for garnish
- Nonstick cooking spray

Direction

1. Using a nonstick spray, spray 4 pieces of foil.

2. Place a fish fillet on each foil.

3. Top with 1/4 cup salsa.

4. Fold foil, crimping edges tightly to seal.

5. Cook on a hot barbecue grill for about 10 minutes.

6. Remove from grill and open foil packet carefully to avoid the hot steam.

7. Serve each fillet with the sauce on

   rice and garnish with lime wedges.

   Enjoy!

Chili Green Beans

Servings: 4

Total Time: 25 Minutes

Calories: 161

Fat: 3.7 g

Protein: 1.5 g

Carbs: 6.9 g

Fiber: 2.5 g

Ingredients and Quantity

- 1 1/2 cup green beans
- 1 red onion, chopped
- 1 red chili pepper, minced
- 1 tsp. hot paprika
- 2 tomatoes, chopped
- 1 tsp. tomato paste

- 1 tsp. black pepper
- 1 tsp. salt
- 1 cup water
- 1 tbsp. olive oil

Direction

1. In the instant pot, mix the green beans with the onion, pepper and the other ingredients and toss.

2. Close and seal the lid. Set Manual mode (High pressure) and cook green beans for 8 minutes.

3. Then allow natural pressure release for 5 minutes.

4. Open the lid and mix up the green beans carefully. Serve and enjoy!

Zucchini Lasagna

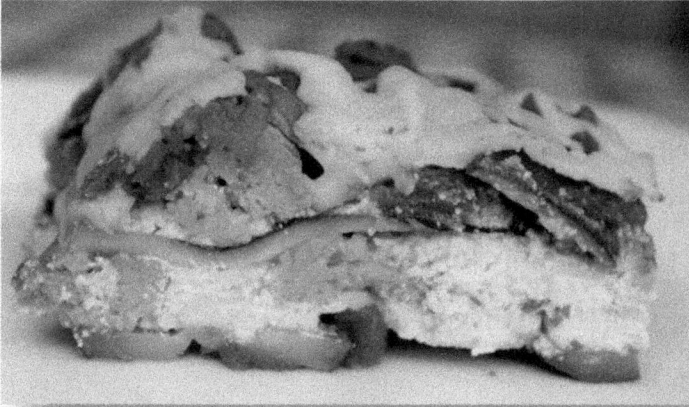

Servings: 2

Total Time: 31 Minutes

Calories: 308

Fat: 13.2 g

Protein: 10.4 g

Carbs: 10.8 g

Fiber: 5.5 g

Ingredients and Quantity

- 3 oz. almonds, crushed
- 1/4 tsp. salt
- 1/2 tsp. black pepper
- 1 tbsp. water
- 1 tsp. olive oil
- 1/2 tsp. lemon juice
- 6 oz. tomatoes, diced and canned
- 3 oz. kale
- 1 zucchini
- 1 tsp. dried oregano
- 1 tsp. Italian seasoning
- 1 onion, grated

Direction

1. In the food processor blend together almonds, salt, water, and olive oil.

2. When the mixture is smooth, transfer it in the mixing bowl.

3. After this, blend lemon juice with diced tomatoes, dried oregano, Italian seasoning, and grated onion.

4. Cut the zucchini lengthwise. The "lasagna" noodles are prepared.

5. Then place little bit tomato mixture in the bottom of the instant pot.

6. Place one zucchini slice and spread it with cashew mixture.

7. Repeat the same steps till you use all the ingredients.

8. Close and seal the lid. Set High-pressure mode and cook the meal for 9 minutes.

9. Then allow natural pressure release for 9 minutes.

10. 10. Open the lid and chill the lasagna till it reaches room temperature. Serve and enjoy!

Ginger Tofu

Servings: 2

Total Time: 20 Minutes

Calories: 261

Fat: 16.9 g

Protein: 22.6 g

Carbs: 10.4 g

Fiber: 2.5 g

Ingredients and Quantity

- 1 pound firm tofu, roughly cubed
- 1 tsp. minced garlic
- 11/2 tsp. minced ginger
- 6 tbsp. soy sauce
- 1 tsp. avocado oil
- 1 tbsp. balsamic vinegar
- 1/2 tsp. brown sugar
- 1/2 tsp. red chili pepper
- 1/4 cup water

Direction

1. In the instant pot, mix the tofu with the garlic, ginger and the other ingredients. Toss gently and close the lid.

2. Set Manual mode (high pressure) and cook a meal for 5 minutes.

3. Make a quick pressure release.

4. Transfer the cooked meal into the serving bowls and top with the gravy. Serve and enjoy!

Tofu and Sauce

Servings: 4

Total Time: 13 Minutes

Calories: 245

Fat: 19.8 g

Protein: 12.8 g

Carbs: 8.4 g

Fiber: 2.9 g

Ingredients and Quantity

- 10 oz. firm tofu, cubed
- 1/4 cup vegetable stock
- 1 tsp. turmeric powder
- 1 tsp. basil, dried
- 1/2 tsp. Salt
- 1 tsp. ground black pepper
- 1 tbsp. avocado oil
- 1/2 tsp. corn flour
- 4 tbsp. coconut butter

- 5 tbsp. almond yogurt
- 1/2 tsp. curry powder
- 1 tbsp. soy sauce
- 1/4 cup peanuts, chopped
- 1/2 tsp. dried rosemary

Direction

1. Sprinkle tofu with salt and place in the instant pot. Add the stock and close the lid.

2. Cook the tofu on High pressure mode for 1 minute.

3. Then use quick pressure release.

4. Add the rest of the ingredients and toss gently.

5. Close and seal the lid. Cook the meal for 2 minutes on Manual mode.

6. Then use quick pressure release.

7. Transfer the tofu into the serving plates and top with gravy. Serve and enjoy!

Lemon Soybeans

Servings: 10

Total Time: 36 Hours

Calories: 125

Fat: 5.6 g

Protein: 10.2 g

Carbs: 8.4 g

Fiber: 2.6 g

Ingredients and Quantity

- 1 1/2 cup soybeans
- 1 tsp. turmeric powder
- 6 cups water
- 1 tbsp. lemon juice
- 1 tsp. tempeh starter
- 1 cup water, for cooking

Direction

1. Place soybeans, turmeric and 5 cups water in the instant pot. Close and seal the lid.

2. Set High-pressure mode and cook soybeans for 45 minutes.

3. Then allow natural pressure release for 30 minutes.

4. Transfer the cooked soybeans in the bowl and sprinkle with lemon juice and tempeh starter.

5. Mix up the soybeans and transfer into the freezer bags. Seal them.

6. Pour the rest of the water in the instant pot.

7. Add sealed freezer bags with soybeans.

8. Close the lid and set "Yogurt" mode.
   Cook tempeh for 15 hours.

9. When the time is over, the tempeh should get the white color.

10. Remove the tempeh from the instant pot and let it rest for hours. Slice it into the servings. Enjoy!